To my beautiful family and
wonderful friends – you all
keep me gratefully alive every
moment of every day.

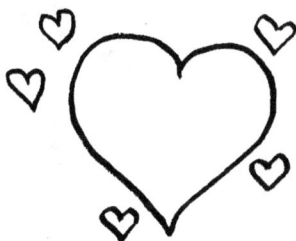

PERPETUALLY PERKY

I am a Stage III breast cancer survivor, so I feel qualified to say that despite the awful negatives of having CANCER, there are also positives. I'm not always perky–well, post-double mastectomy I guess I am, at least on the outside in the boob region. Of course there are times when I have a negative head; that's normal. But Cancer usually becomes the star of the pity party and definitely kicks it into high gear.

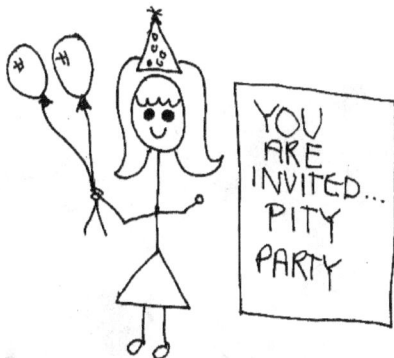

Eventually, though, the pity party has to end; you have to send the blues packing, the wahs and woes need to go home, and the anger has to take a chill pill. It's time to get your head around the big-C and put things back in perspective so you can walk forward happily on your path in life. No, not walk – skip, sing, dance. And yeah, you have to trudge through some muck at first. But even trudging can be positive – if just to appreciate the wonderfulness of a plain old non-trudging day and to be grateful to be alive.

So here are some positives:

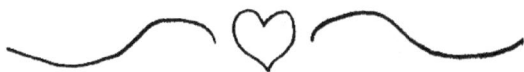

You will forever have perky perfect boobs. If your natural boobs were starting to sag, if they hung so low that you could tuck them into your waistband, or if they gave you a black eye when you were running braless, no worries anymore!

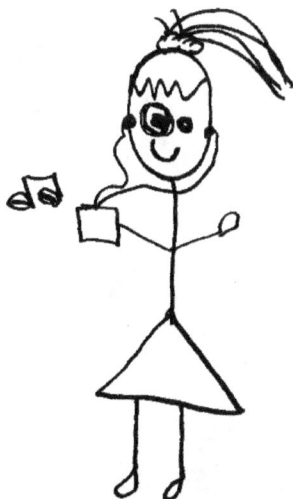

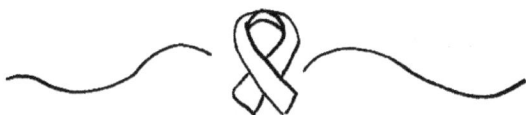

When you have parts surgically removed, you automatically weigh less. And if you end up with prosthetics in your bra rather than implants, it's easy to take off your shoes and bra before stepping on the scale.

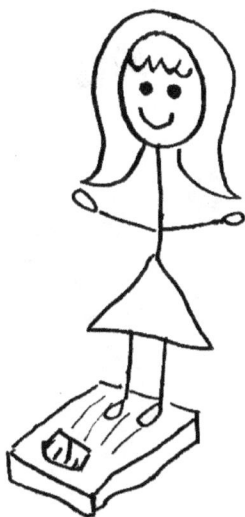

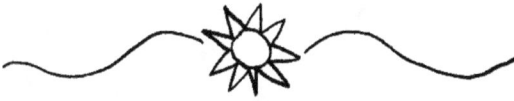

When you are going through chemo, you save a lot of time because you don't have to get haircuts or blow-dry your hair. There's no hair gel, color, mousse, or spray to buy, and you are touted as an environmentalist for taking such quick showers and saving water.

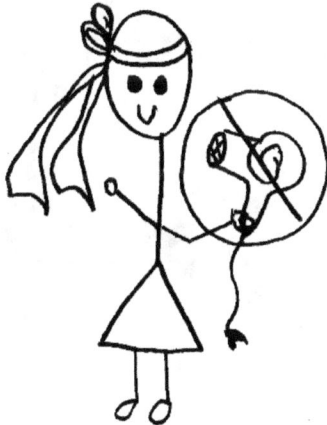

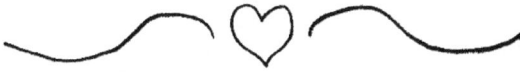

With no hair, you don't have to worry whether your haircut is outdated or not. Bald is bald. Whether it's in or it's out, it just is what it is.

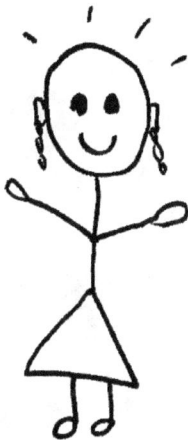

BALD
IS
BEAUTIFUL

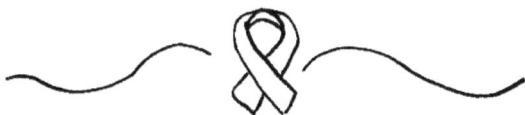

We are all going to have some health problems – no one has figured out immortality just yet. The thing about breast cancer is that there are so many new treatments and ways to fight it. At least there's something to pin hopes on, whether it's for a bit longer or for a cure.

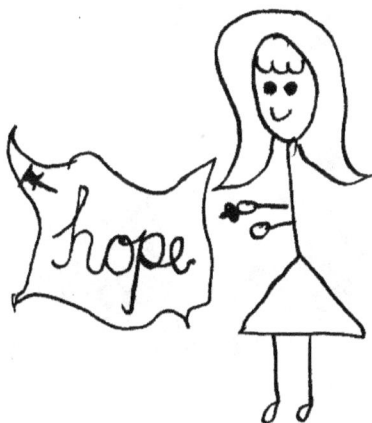

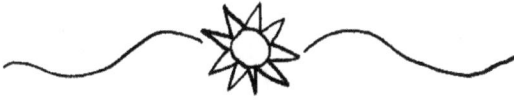

When you are in the hospital or in oncology areas, you see other cancer patients, and you know what strength is. You see what endurance and hope are. You can hear the clink of their invisible armor as they head off to kill their opponent in the infusion room.

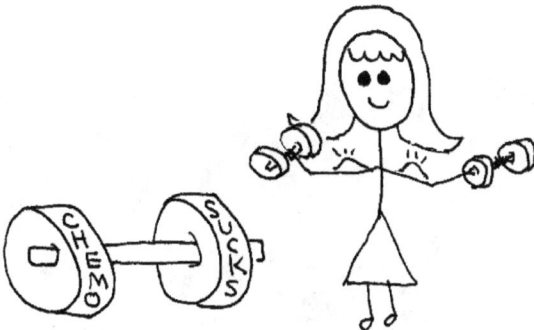

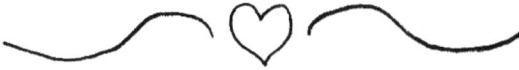

Chemo is a great time to try out wearing hats, which is sort of vogue. Most of us don't walk around every day stylin' in hats; we just don't have that type of fashion sense or pizzazz. But here's your chance – turbans, a knit snow hat, baseball cap, or big floppy hat – anything goes!

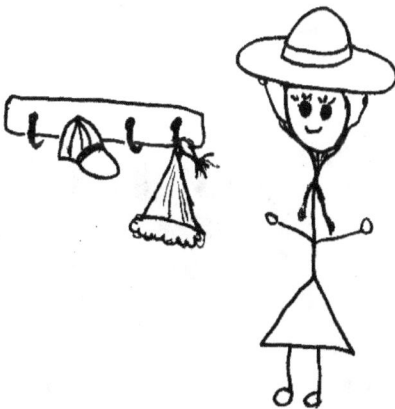

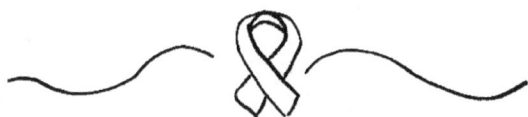

Cancer is a great excuse to get out of those bad social obligations that you know you have to go to but you just totally don't want to. Not even a problem that it's the last minute. Completely excused, no hard feelings.

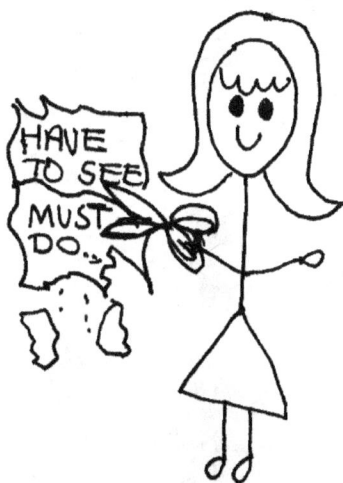

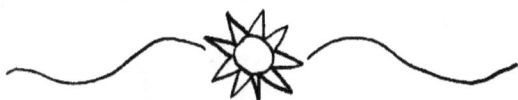

There's no guilt from not working out. You can justify it cuz the big-C process makes you tired. And when you do workout, you feel like a super-athlete. You have cancer AND you worked out – amazing!

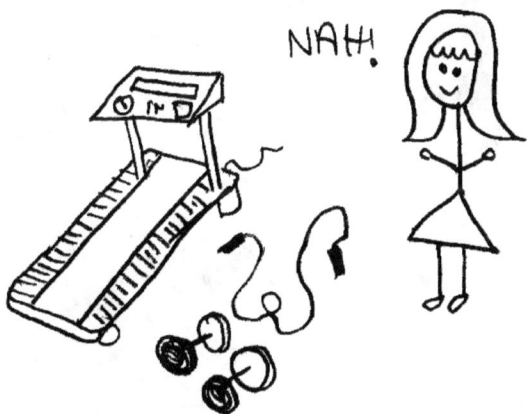

NAH!

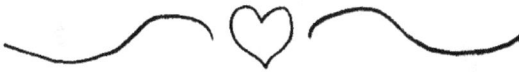

One of the perks of cancer treatments is that you become an amazing sleeper. Whether you are just worn out or it's the medication, you crash before your eyes are even closed. For a non-sleeper who typically spends hours tossing and turning, it's a very nice experience.

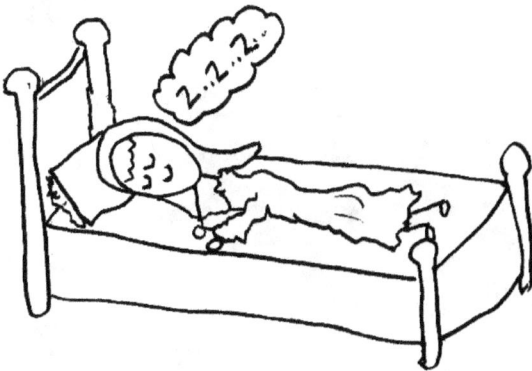

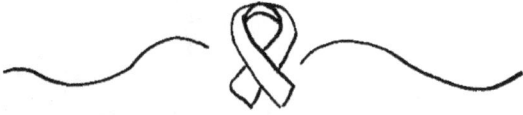

When you have breast cancer, you can have a boob party to celebrate a milestone – including boob-shaped pastry holders and napkins, decorating cupcakes to look like boobs, making little appetizers and other boobular-looking food. And of course have a supply of those candies – "nips."

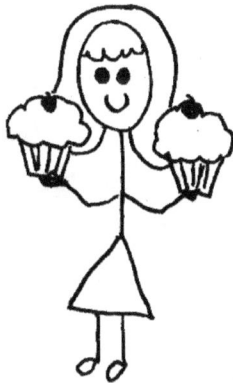

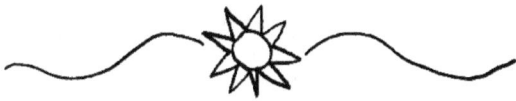

You may be bald, but when your hair grows back you can try out every hair length! You can have the short-hair-career-woman-'do, the getting-longer-fun-sassy-style, or the totally-long-free-spirit-look.

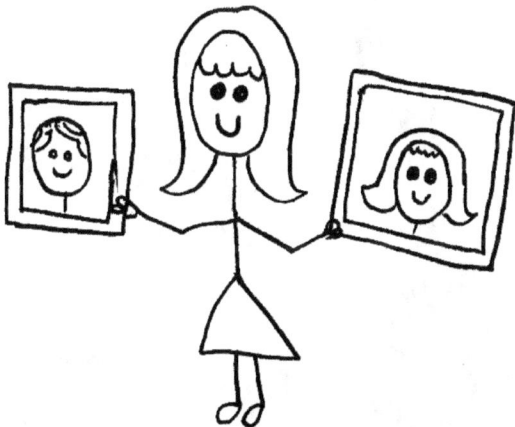

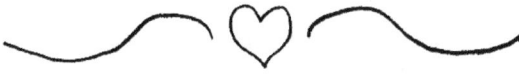

After what you have gone through, many of the annoyances in daily life are no longer bothersome – road rage from an endless traffic jam? Three price checks in a row at the grocery line you are in? Bring it on! Who cares?

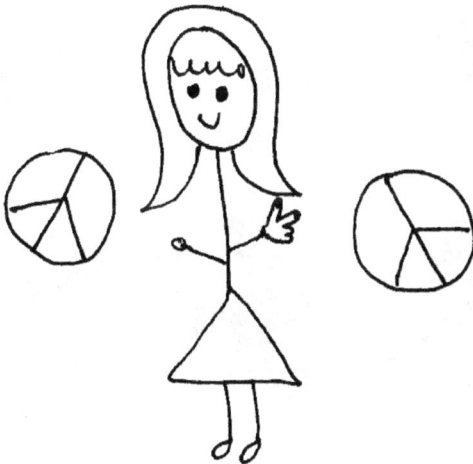

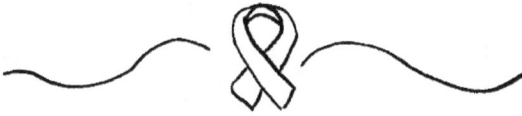

It's a nice perk to have new Goldilocks boobs - not too big and not too small, not too saggy but not too pert, not too lumpy and not too firm, not too high and not too low. They are just right!

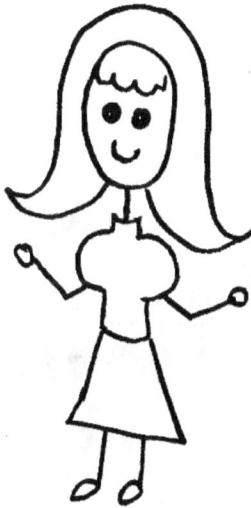

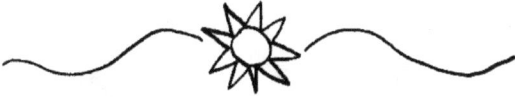

If you have always been grossed out by blood and medical things, cancer is a great way to get over that. After dealing with the nasty post-surgery drains and being stuck with needles endlessly, your medical grossness tolerance really goes up!

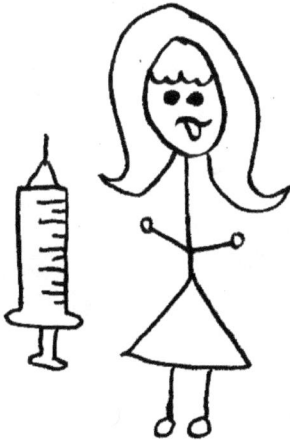

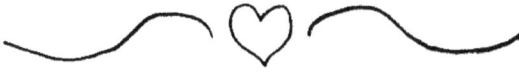

You are strong; you are as solid as a brick wall. And Cancer, like the big bad wolf, can't get to you. Yeah, maybe it will mess up your outside shell a little, but it's not going to mess up your inside serenity and positive 'tude. Cancer is just a big dumb blow-hard, like the wolf.

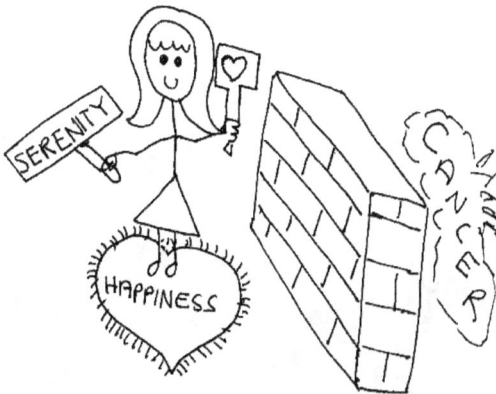

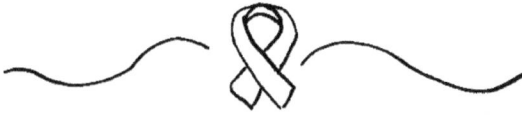

When you get those funky mouth sores from the chemo, you really can't eat your low-cal grapefruit – better to stick with smooth, cooling ice cream. Of course the sprinkles and hot fudge sauce on top are not necessary but how else can you FORCE down the ice cream?!

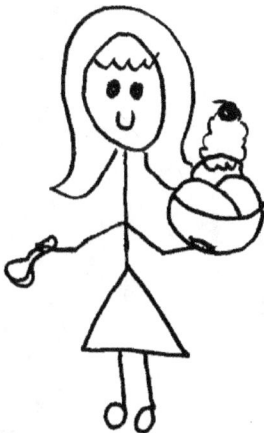

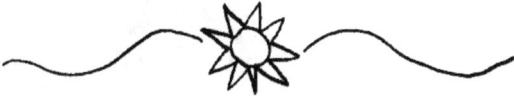

You get out of a lot of chores during that time period of having surgeries, radiation, chemo, and more surgeries. You are too tired, can't lift more than five pounds, not supposed to drive. Whatever the situation calls for, you can pull out an applicable medical restriction.

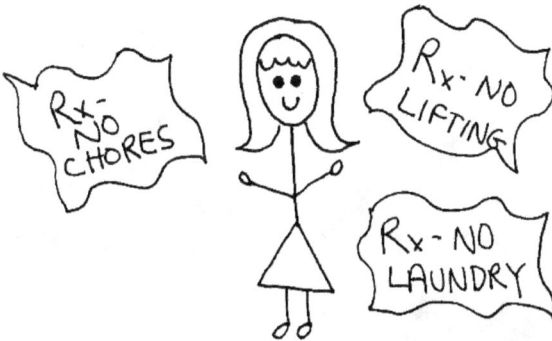

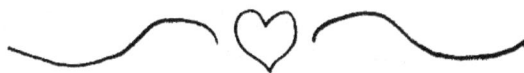

Slippers – a big gift item. Before you are done, chances are you will have multi-colored slippers, bear claw slippers, kitty slippers, slippers with heels, slide-in slippers, bootie slippers, flip-flop slippers, ultra-thick fuzzy sock-type slippers, and of course pink slippers.

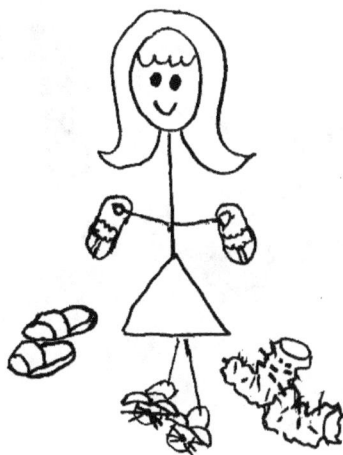

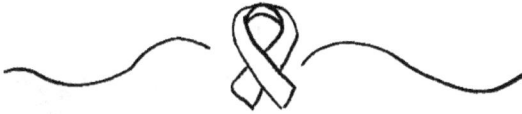

Your never-ending, years-old to-do list is completed – the tasks either get done without any more nagging or they get removed from the list because you realize it's not worth wasting time on. What a freeing feeling!

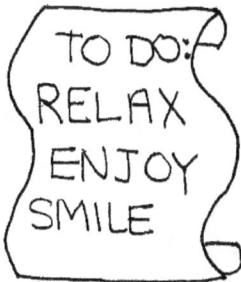

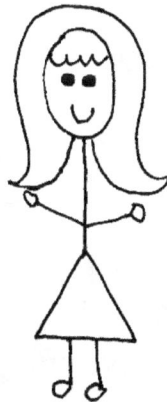

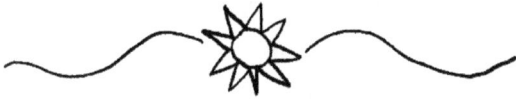

It's probably not your most attractive look to be bald, but it's also not attractive to wake up with bed hair, have a totally uncontrolled frizzy hair day, or have a completely flat, no-body hair day.

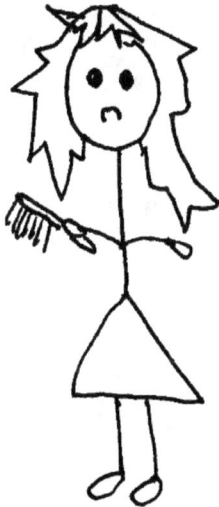

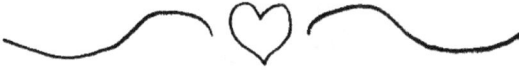

When you get the cancer diagnosis, chances are it's one of the worst moments in your life. And that's sort of reassuring to get it over with. There will be other bad things - but you already know you have inner strength to handle it because you went through your hardest time.

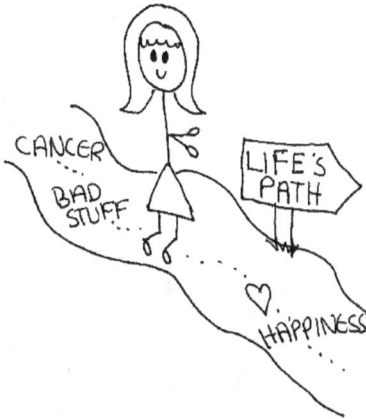

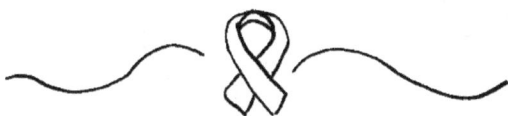

If you like to swim or just splash around in the water, your implants are your own personal floaters. You won't ever have to worry about drowning – those things double as buoyancy safety devices – nice!

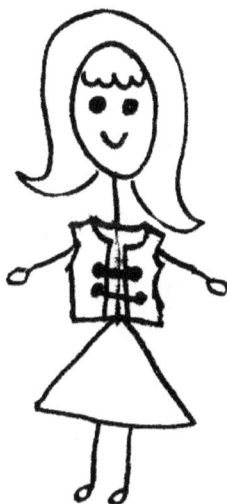

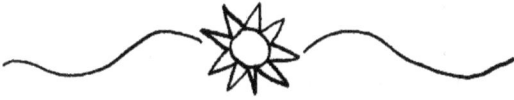

You get to throw around remarks like, "Yes, I have a couple tattoos." Thanks Radiation Markers! There is also the tattooed area for the reconstruction – some women want it to look real, others go for the flower or heart shape. Cancer survivors are hip!

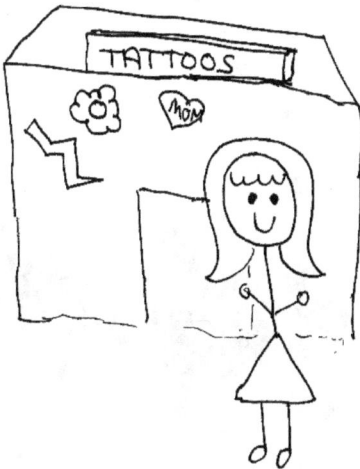

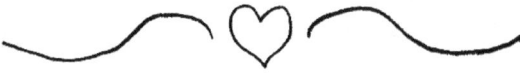

People constantly tell you
how much courage you
have and how brave you
are. Well, you deal with
what you have to, what's
the choice? All the same,
it's really strengthening to
hear it.

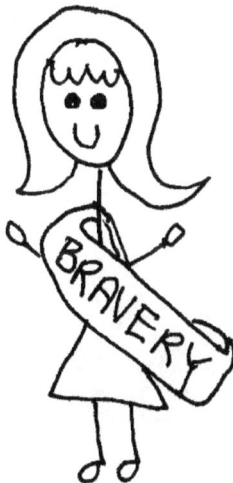

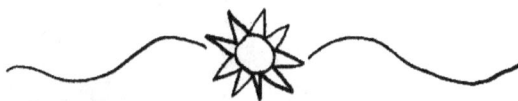

When someone pulls a
gross, disgusting long hair
out of the food on the
dinner table, there's no
way it can be blamed on
you!

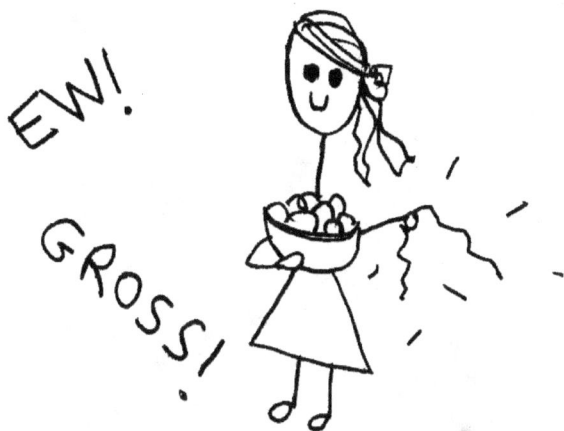

EW!

GROSS!

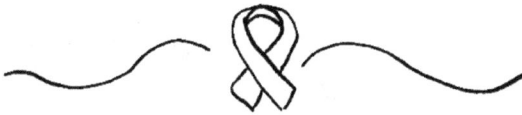

When you go through the Big-C, other C-Club members know you are a member, too. You might be shopping with a snow hat over your bald head, a stranger comes over and says, "I was there six years ago. You will get past it," and then gives you a hug and walks away. The words are so strengthening; the hug is everything.

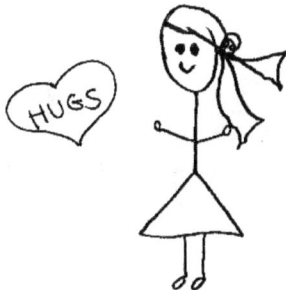

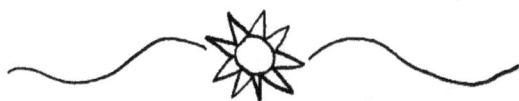

Implants work like football players' padding – impact is greatly reduced. Next time you get elbowed in a crowd or the person next to you in the kickboxing class throws a kick that ends up being too close, no worries.

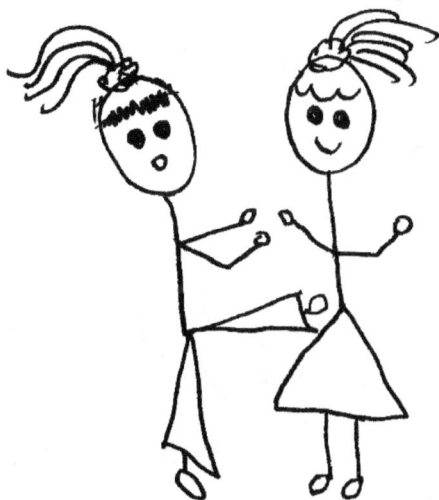

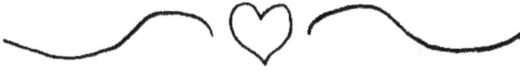

The friendships you make along the way with other warriors are steel-strong bonds because it's the real thing, totally intense. Not in the same league as dissing a preschool teacher, whining about carpool lines, or griping about grocery prices. Amazingly, there are a lot of laughs even while the toxic mixture is being infused.

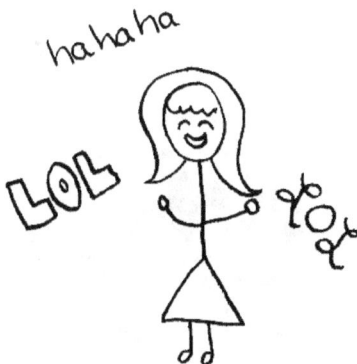

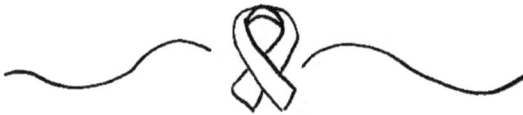

You need more dresser space for all your new PJs and robes. You get them as gifts, and since you have Cancer, you get the plushest, silkiest, and cutest bedtime wear. No more wearing sweat pants and a stained, partly ripped, old t-shirt to bed!

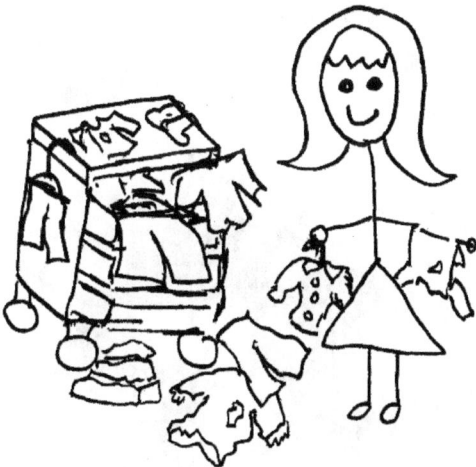

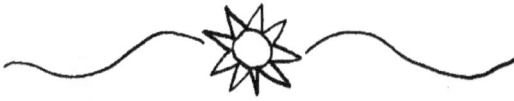

You can swear when you want to and people don't judge you or think you are a hussy. It's okay to describe cancer with every bad word you've ever heard, and any string of them together that you can make.

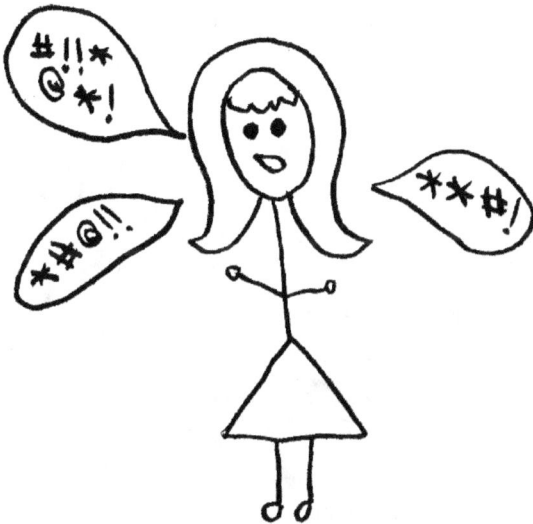

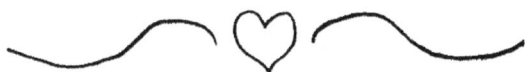

You can ride in a convertible or on a motorcycle and not worry about that wind-blown hair look – because you are either bald from the chemo, or your post-chemo hair is too bristly and frizzy to move.

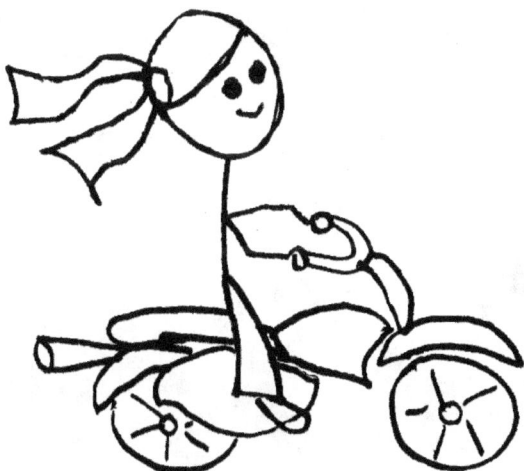

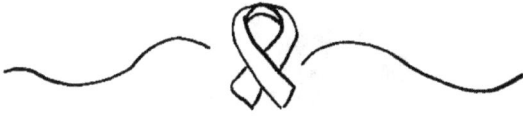

Chemo brain – it's a real thing. So is spaciness. But one is respected and one isn't so much. When you lock your keys in the car, lose your grocery list, or forget someone's name – you finally have a legitimate excuse.

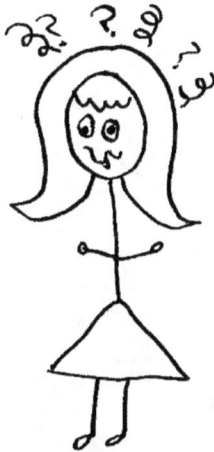

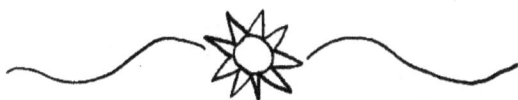

If your husband or kids cook something for you, luckily you lose your sense of taste a little so you don't have to worry about their use of 2 tablespoons of cayenne powder instead of ½ teaspoon, or doing a pour instead of a dash of salt.

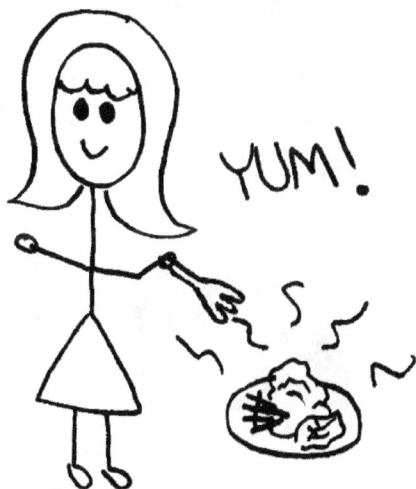

YUM!

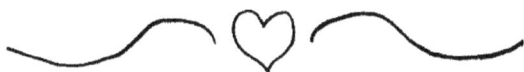

When you find out you have cancer, chances are you lose your appetite and lose some weight. You have surgery and lose a little more. Radiation and chemo take their toll and you might lose a bit more weight. Having cancer is not a fad diet, but you certainly shed pounds without effort. Perk!

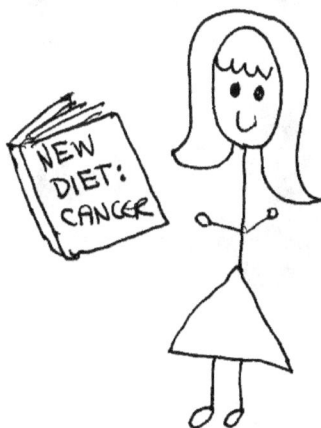

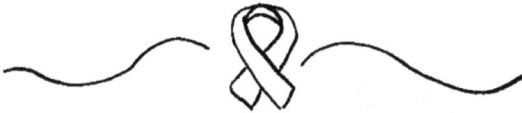

If you cry easily at Disney movies or your kid's play, people now chalk it up to surviving the big-C and they "totally understand." You gotta love those built-in excuses for your normal personality glitches.

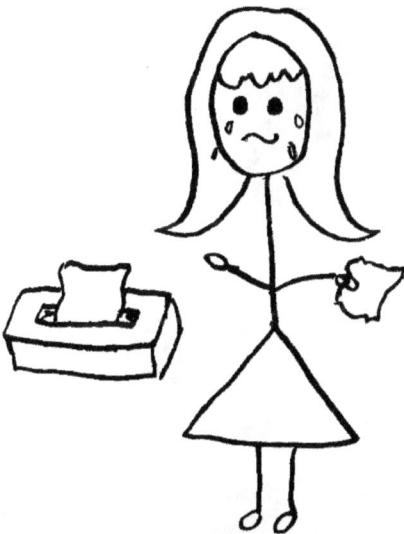

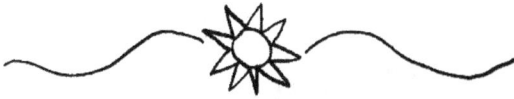

There's no need to shave. No mascara to put on. No eyebrows to pluck or shape. When you tell the kids you are jumping in the shower and will be ready to go in 10 minutes, you really mean 8 minutes instead of the previous 45 minutes.

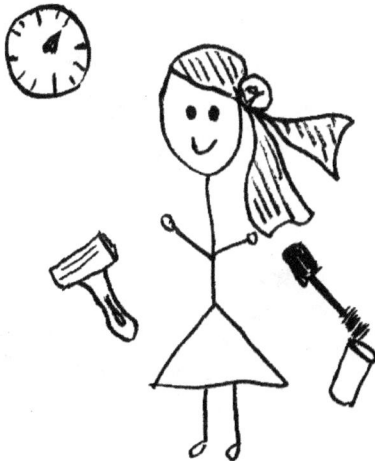

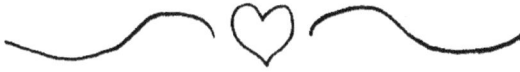

When you are having those long chemo sessions, you have plenty of time to do fun arts and crafts projects, like coloring. Bring paper, markers, and colored pencils and you'll be the hit of the infusion center!

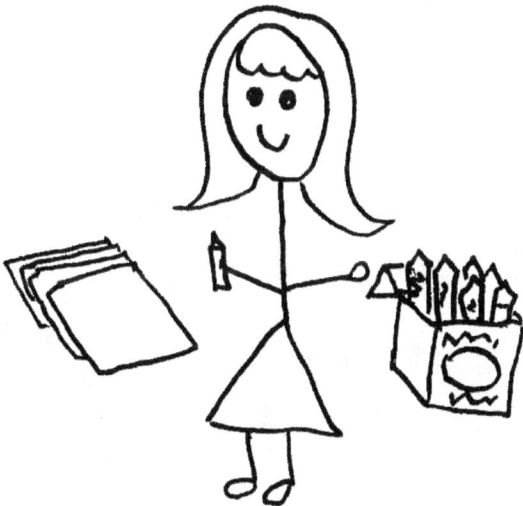

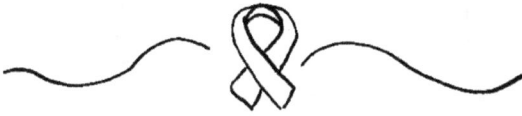

Radiation may be a pain in the butt because it's daily, but on the flip side, if you don't finish a magazine article you are reading, it's there the next day for you to continue. You never miss an issue of People magazine and are completely in the know about Brad and Angelina.

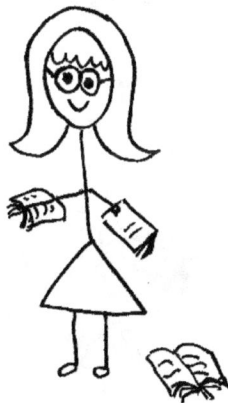

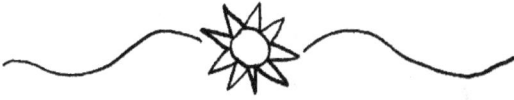

Pink is an easy color to wear and a pretty color to have a lot of stuff in, so that's lucky. If you had a cancer that had an ugly color associated with it, you'd be bummed out with a lot of ugly colored things.

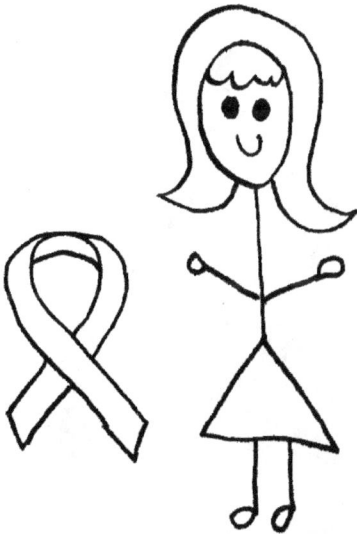

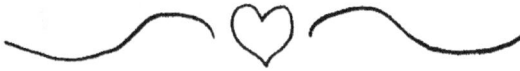

You really get to know
who your friends are.
They are the ones who are
there spiritually 24/7, but
respect that you might
need your space. They
drive you around and
don't get a free lunch out
of it. They are uplifting,
positive, and ready to
party for any celebratory
milestone. They are there
for you through thick and
thin (as in hair, body, and
life moments).

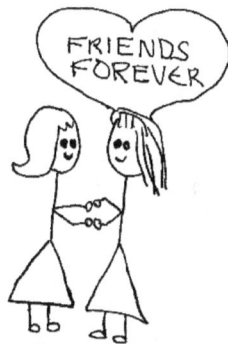

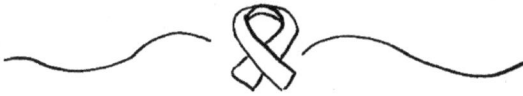

And family – new bonds are made, strong bonds are strengthened. They run interference from nosy relatives who ask too many questions, and remind you that "we are family" while singing that hokey tune. The shared tears are so deep and intense - celebrations so heightened with giddiness and appreciation of life.

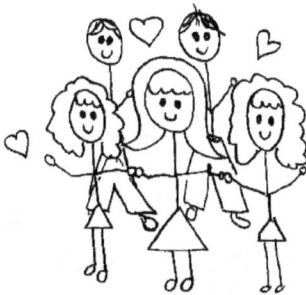

WE ARE FAMILY

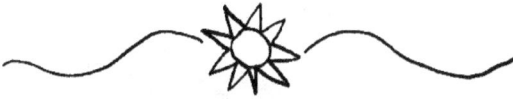

It's the support from those in your life that makes the tough times manageable; whether it's family, old friends, new chemo buddies – we are all here to help one another – to remind each other that there are always dark clouds before the rainbows. You will get through this. Dancing is around the corner.

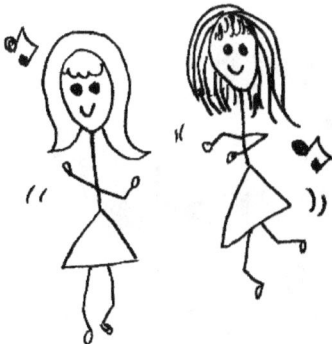

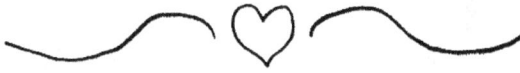

Because anyway, cancer
sucks. It's a bitch, it's
mean. No one likes you,
Cancer, so just get the
hell out of here. We are
slamming the door behind
you, Cancer. And locking
it. You aren't welcome
here. Screw you, Cancer.

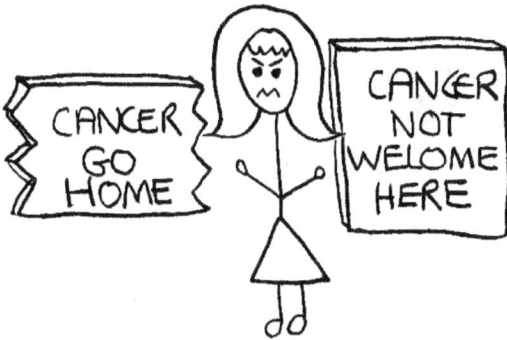

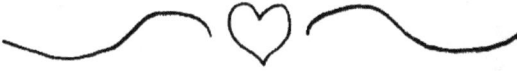

AND REMEMBER – when you are done with your stuff – your hats, your turbans, your former bras, donate them! Even old prosthetics that you have updated to more perky ones can find a new chest to rest on for people whose insurance does not cover them.

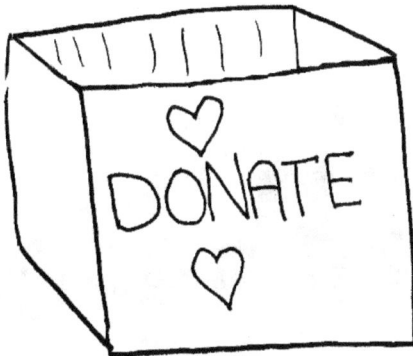